Safe Sedation, Analgesia and Anaesthesia within the Radiology Department

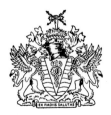

Board of Faculty of Clinical Radiology
The Royal College of Radiologists

The Royal College of Radiologists
38 Portland Place
London W1B 1JQ

Telephone 020 7636 4432
Fax 020 7323 3100

Citation details:
Board of Faculty of Clinical Radiology
The Royal College of Radiologists (2003)
Safe Sedation, Analgesia and Anaesthesia
within the Radiology Department
Royal College of Radiologists, London.
Email: enquiries@rcr.ac.uk
On publication this document will be made
available on the College's web site: http://
www.rcr.ac.uk

ISBN 1872599 91 5

BFCR(03)4

Design and print: Intertype:www.intertype.co.uk

Contents

Foreword

Concerns have been raised about the safety of sedation techniques used for healthcare procedures by different specialty groups and that guidance on the safe use of sedative drugs is often not followed, either through lack of awareness, lack of training or insufficient staff due to financial constraints, leading to exposure to unnecessary risk. All Colleges have been asked by the Academy of Medical Royal Colleges to review the position for their specialities. This document represents the Royal College of Radiologists' attempt to establish safe guidance for radiology departments on analgesics and anaesthetics in addition to sedation. Whilst sedation techniques, together with good pain relief and sympathetic patient management can make certain healthcare procedures more acceptable to patients, patients should not be exposed to unnecessary risk and patient safety must be preserved.

The environment within which radiology is delivered becomes ever more complex, and radiologists deliver an increasingly varied range of procedures. Frequently resource issues are at the heart of the capacity of departments to fulfil the demands placed on them, but safe and effective practice must be paramount. Good access to anaesthetics for radiology is vital, as is provision for adequate monitoring during radiology procedures performed under sedation. I hope the document provides an overview of the issues, accepting that the total care package inevitably comprises a wider range of issues, and that it will assist departments in reviewing their policies and those responsible for commissioning healthcare to ensure that safe practices are in place.

I would like to thank the members of the working party who prepared this document on behalf of the Faculty:

Juliet Britton, consultant neuroradiologist, Atkinson Morley's Hospital, Wimbledon

Alastair Chalmers, consultant radiologist, Royal United Hospital, Bath (chairman)

Derrick Martin, consultant radiologist, South Manchester University Hospital, Manchester

Kieran McHugh, consultant paediatric radiologist, Great Ormond Street Hospital for Children, London

Lizete Pearson, senior clinical nurse, Southampton University Hospital, Southampton

Carol Peden, consultant anaesthetist, Royal United Hospital, Bath

Monica Stokes, consultant paediatric anaesthetist, Birmingham Childrens' Hospital, Birmingham

Particular thanks are due to the Alastair Chalmers for his work as chairman. I would also like to acknowledge the help of all of the individuals who provided advice, in particular: Dr Stephen L. Hill (consultant anaesthetist, Royal United Hospital, Bath); Dr Mike Sury, consultant anaesthetist, Hospital for Sick Children, London; and members of the RCR Interventional Radiology Subcommittee.

Dr Mike Dean
Dean
Faculty of Clinical Radiology

Executive Summary

1. The Medical Royal Colleges have been requested by the Academy of Medical Royal Colleges to produce specialty-specific guidance regarding the use of sedation, analgesia and anaesthesia. This document contains generic guidance for departments of clinical radiology in the use of these techniques and specific guidance for the subspecialties of paediatric, cross-sectional and adult interventional radiology.

2. Large increases in the number and scope of procedures performed in radiology departments have taken place since 1992 when the last College guidelines on Sedation and Anaesthesia[1] were produced.

3. Sedation is only part of a 'package' of care comprising pre-assessment, properly informed consent, adequate facilities, good techniques and risk avoidance.

4. 'Heavy', 'conscious' or 'deep' sedation are unsatisfactory and misleading terms and should not be used in adult practice. In paediatrics a deeper level of sedation is acceptable, is strictly defined, and should be administered only by an anaesthetist or other appropriately trained healthcare professional.

5. If an adult patient is sedated to a point where they are unrousable to verbal or painless physical stimuli, then that patient is anaesthetised, not sedated, with all the inherent risks attached.

6. The recommended facilities for the safe administration of sedation and analgesia are defined in other publications[1-4] and include piped oxygen, pulse oximetry, electrocardiography, automated blood pressure/pulse measurement and the availability of resuscitation equipment and reversal agents.

7. Radiology departments need adequate space for pre-assessment and recovery. Ideally, this should all be within the radiology department.

8. Ideally the patient should be monitored by a healthcare professional, trained to administer sedation who will not have any other role at the time of the procedure. It is difficult for the radiologist performing the procedure to safely monitor the patient unaided.

9. Providing staff to monitor a patient is currently a difficult area for many departments. The overriding consideration must be that patient safety should not be compromised because of staffing or financial constraints.

10. Some non-vascular interventional procedures can cause severe pain and require sedation and analgesia administered by an appropriately trained healthcare professional with the appropriate level of monitoring.

11. There are some procedures that radiologists might consider require general anaesthetic, because they are particularly painful or because of the individual needs of a particular patient. If such anaesthetic support is not available then it might be inappropriate to perform that procedure.

12. Due to the increasing complexity of many radiological procedures, including those in the young and very elderly, a greater need for anaesthetic assistance and sessions in radiology departments should be anticipated.

13. Many radiologists already have extensive experience in administering sedation and analgesia but in the future formal training in sedation and anaesthesia techniques should be part of an interventional radiology training programme. Training and examination in the principles and practice of sedation, analgesia and resuscitation are necessary for all radiologists. Refresher lectures should be incorporated into general and specialty radiology meetings and courses.

14. A healthy relationship with the anaesthetic department is clearly useful to facilitate the provision of complex sedation and general anaesthesia. Radiology and anaesthetic departments should co-operate in the training programmes of each other's juniors so that each understands the requirements and limitations of the other, and to foster good relations and working practices. Audit of process and outcomes relating to sedation and analgesia should be regularly undertaken to ensure quality and promote reflective practice.

1 Introduction

1.1   In July 1992 the Royal Colleges of Radiologists and Anaesthetists produced advice entitled *Sedation and Anaesthesia in Radiology*.[1] Since then great changes have taken place in radiology departments in terms of the number and scope of the procedures performed. Complex radiological techniques, some of which are painful, are widely practised.

1.2   In November 2001 the Academy of Medical Royal Colleges published the report of a working party entitled *Implementing and Ensuring Safe Sedation Practice for Healthcare Procedures in Adults*.[2] It reviewed existing guidelines relating to sedation for healthcare procedures and charged Royal Colleges and other organisations with the responsibility for developing specialty-specific guidance.

1.3   The Scottish Intercollegiate Guidelines Network produced a national clinical guideline entitled *Safe Sedation of Children Undergoing Diagnostic and Therapeutic Procedures* in 2002[3] and the Association of Anaesthetists of Great Britain and Ireland published *Provision of Anaesthetic Services in Magnetic Resonance Units*.[4]

1.4   'It is no longer appropriate for the operator/anaesthetist role to be borne by the interventional radiologist alone'.[5] It is clear that there is no shortage of advice from various quarters relating to sedation and anaesthesia in radiology. In response to the Academy of Medical Royal Colleges and the need to revise their existing advice, the Royal College of Radiologists established a multidisciplinary working party to produce an updated document providing advice for radiologists and their departments.

1.5   The working party has brought together information from a variety of sources, and this document is intended to provide guidance regarding analgesia, sedation and anaesthesia for patients having examinations in radiology departments. It is hoped that users will find it to be a practical guide regarding equipment, facilities, staffing and pharmacology. It also covers the issues of training, audit and revalidation.

1.6   It is important to realise that sedation, analgesia or anaesthesia when required are only part of a 'package' of care comprising good information, informed consent, adequate facilities, risk avoidance and good technique. Although this document concentrates on sedation, analgesia and anaesthesia, these other areas are integral.

1.7   The requirements of subspecialties such as interventional radiology, cross-sectional imaging and paediatrics differ considerably. This document consists mainly of general points which should be read by all users, but also provides additional information applicable to other radiology subspecialties.

1.8   Whilst there are details on drugs and dosages in the paediatric section (Section 11.1), these have not been included in the other sub-specialty sections because of drug interactions and the rapidity with which such advice goes out of date. The drugs listed in the paediatric section are for guidance only, and some individuals may choose to give alternatives.

2 Interdepartmental Co-operation

2.1   Good relationships between a hospital's department of radiology and department of anaesthesia are key to providing the best environment for good working practices. Relationships have to be fostered in a spirit of mutual understanding, bearing in mind resource limitations and other problems. The following points should be considered:

- departments should identify a person to manage the cooperation;
- radiologists should invite anaesthetists to their department to show them the current scope of work;
- anaesthetic departments should be involved in the training of junior radiologists;
- there should be liaison over the production of local protocols;
- there should be an agreed plan for the management of unexpected emergencies in a radiology department;
- fixed anaesthetic sessions in radiology may be satisfactory in some departments but a more flexible arrangement may be more efficient where the demand is unpredictable;
- the paediatric and neuroradiology requirements for sedation, analgesia and anaesthesia need to be considered when planning anaesthetic services. If departments with other specialized services require anaesthetic support frequently enough to demand such consideration, then clearly anaesthetic services should take these into account also.

2.2   The quality of cooperation between the departments should be assessed in 'training and accreditation' visits by the respective Royal Colleges.

3 Techniques

3.1 Analgesia

3.1.1   Analgesia is the control of pain. Pain is a spectrum. The need for analgesia is reduced if the patient is comfortable and has confidence in the radiology team.[6]

3.1.2   Analgesic drug doses should be given incrementally and the minimum dose used so that the patient remains rousable. Initially, analgesics should be given before sedatives to reduce the risk of respiratory depression.

3.2 Anaesthesia

Anaesthesia can be local, general, regional, or spinal/epidural.

3.2.1   Local anaesthesia

For all percutaneous techniques local anaesthesia should be used irrespective of the use of sedation and analgesia. Even for some general anaesthetic regimens it may be appropriate to use local anaesthesia. Lignocaine 1 or 2% is the agent of choice. Following the procedure longer acting local anaesthetic agents may be used, e.g., Bupivicaine 0.5%. Inadvertent intravascular injection of local anaesthetics must be avoided as this can be life threatening.

Radiologists should be familiar with the use of local anaesthetics, know advised maximum doses and be competent in the management of complications.

For patients with a particular aversion to percutaneous punctures a topical local anaesthetic cream can be used.

3.2.2   General anaesthesia

Performing general anaesthesia in a radiology department may have some additional hazards compared to working in an operating theatre:

- poor access to the patient during the procedure;
- unfamiliar environment/equipment;
- dim lighting;
- noise and distractions;
- remote location from anaesthetic services and recovery facilities.

A radiologist should not administer general anaesthetics or give drugs in a dosage which may produce general anaesthesia.

'The x-ray department is a more difficult environment than the operating theatre in which to give an anaesthetic. It is, therefore, inappropriate for an inexperienced anaesthetist to be responsible for such cases.'[7] If an anaesthetist is required there should also be an operating department/anaesthetic assistant present.

3.2.3   Regional anaesthesia

For some procedures regional anaesthetic techniques, for example interpleural block or paraspinal block, may be appropriate. It is not unreasonable for radiologists to use these techniques themselves provided they are properly trained in the technique and the management of any complication.

3.2.4   Spinal or epidural anaesthesia

These techniques are used extensively for obstetrics, intra-abdominal, hip and leg surgery, but until the last few years have been little used in radiology. Radiologists should discuss with their local anaesthetists whether such methods may be helpful in their practice.

3.3 Sedation

3.3.1 Sedation is 'a technique in which the use of a drug or drugs produces a state of depression of the central nervous system enabling treatment to be carried out, but during which verbal contact with the patient is maintained throughout the period of sedation. The drugs and techniques used should carry a margin of safety wide enough to render unintended loss of consciousness unlikely'.[8] For the definition in children see the paediatric subspecialty section (Section 11.1).

3.3.2 If all verbal contact is lost and the patient becomes unrousable to painless physical stimuli, then that patient is anaesthetised, not sedated, with all the inherent risks attached.

3.3.3 Most patients are anxious before a diagnostic or interventional procedure particularly if they are in pain. A pre-procedure visit with friendly support and explanation in the radiology department reduces the need for sedation. Sedatives should be offered if anxiety persists or if the patient would feel more comfortable during a procedure.

3.3.4 If the procedure is being done on a day case or outpatient basis sedatives can be prescribed at the pre-assessment visit, to be taken on the day of the examination.

3.3.5 The most popular drugs for intravenous use are Midazolam or Diazepam in aqueous solution. Diazepam in oily solution (Valium) is thrombogenic and is no longer recommended. The dose of benzodiazepines is titrated to the patient's needs remembering that at least 2 min should pass after intravenous injection for the effect to be assessed and before a further dose is given. The amnesic effects of benzodiazepines are greater than the sedative effects. Midazolam is preferable to Diazepam since it has a much shorter half-life.

3.3.6 Sedation, like analgesia, should be given incrementally so that consciousness is not lost or respiration depressed. Sedation should not be used as a replacement for analgesia and if both are required the analgesic drugs should be given first because of possible synergistic effects.

3.3.7 It may be necessary to top up the dose of opioid in a sedated patient if a particularly painful manoeuvre during the procedure is anticipated (for example biliary stricture dilatation). Such painful procedures are particularly problematic. The level of sedation and analgesia needs to be higher than with many other interventional radiological manoeuvres. While discouraging the use of the concept and term 'deep' sedation, it is recognised that these patients frequently need to be heavily sedated. As long as patients are still rousable to verbal command or painless physical stimuli they are sedated and not anaesthetised.

3.3.8 Outpatients receiving either oral or intravenous sedation need to be accompanied to the department by a friend or relative. They need to be advised that having received sedation the patient should not drive for 24 h. This should also be stated in the information sheet. The ability to drive may be impaired for up to 48 h following the use of Diazepam.

3.3.9 Patients who are to receive intravenous sedation must undergo a period of fasting the same as if they were having a general anaesthetic, i.e., 6 h for solid food and milk, 2 h for clear fluids e.g., water, black coffee or black tea.

3.4 Oxygen usage

3.4.1 Respiratory depression occurs with intravenous analgesic and sedative drugs and more so with combinations. Hypoxia can occur. The administration of oxygen at 2–4 l/min via nasal cannulae can abolish hypoxia in most patients. If intravenous opioid or benzodiazepines or a combination is anticipated, pre-oxygenation must be given prior to intravenous drug administration and maintained throughout the period of the procedure and recovery.

3.4.2 The SpO_2 (soluble partial pressure of oxygen) should be measured with a pulse oximeter throughout a procedure when sedation, analgesia or anaesthesia is used. Measurement can cease when recovery criteria are met. (See Section 6—Monitoring.)

3.5 Drugs

3.5.1 Maintenance of an adequate range of analgesic, sedative, anaesthetic and resuscitative drugs should be the responsibility of the lead radiology nurse, advised and assisted by radiologists, anaesthetists and the hospital pharmacy. Expiry dates of drugs should be checked monthly by a designated person.

3.5.2 Drug cupboards easily accessible to all areas where analgesia, sedation and anaesthesia are undertaken are required. This may mean having more than one.

3.5.3 Clear, legible labelling of drugs is required. Some preparations have tiny lettering on labels and operators need to take particular care with this inherent risk. Additional colour coding can reduce this problem. A protocol by which a particular size of syringe is used for an agreed substance (e.g., contrast medium, saline, anaesthetic) is used in some departments as a further safety measure.

3.5.4 Specific antagonists for intravenously used drugs must be immediately available. The availability of specific antagonists should not encourage the overuse of intravenous analgesic or sedative drugs. They should not be used to hasten discharge. Antagonists should be prominently labelled and indicate against which drug they are effective.

3.5.5 It is important to keep the perceived level of risk from sedation and analgesia in proportion to the potential benefits. Radiologists should maintain their Advanced Techniques of Life Support skills in order to deal with complications and they should have ready access to a crash call system.

4 Pre-assessment

4.1 General

4.1.1 Assessment of the patient before the procedure should be standard practice. The development of care pathways enables this to be integral to the planning of a procedure. Pre-assessment enables the physical and mental state of the patient to be assessed as both of these may have altered since the request for the procedure was made. It enables a member of the radiology team to assess the likely level of sedation or analgesia that will be required, if any. This is particularly important before interventional procedures. Time to undertake pre-assessment and the consent process should be built into radiologists' job plans.

4.1.2 Information regarding the procedure can be given to the patient. This can be in the form of leaflets, e.g., from the RCR website (www.rcr.ac.uk.), locally produced videos and/or discussion. The more understanding there is about a procedure, the less the anxiety.[6] Questions can be answered and consent obtained.

4.2 Day cases

4.2.1 Patients intended for a daycase procedure, whether using sedation or not, should have the following assessed:

- access to living accommodation;
- distance from the hospital;
- presence of responsible adult at home;
- transport arrangements;
- telephone availability.

4.2.2 Before leaving the pre-assessment the patient should be sure of the following:

- time of arrival to radiology department/hospital;
- when to fast from if necessary;
- what drugs can be taken if fasting. Generally all routine drugs excluding insulin, oral hypoglycaemics and anticoagulants, should be taken as usual on the day of the procedure with a sip of water. Cardiovascular medication and regular analgesics should be taken where appropriate. Local protocols should be developed for the management of fasting diabetic patients;
- contact names and telephone numbers of someone knowledgeable within the department who can answer further questions.

4.3 Ward patients

Inpatients coming to radiology departments for procedures requiring sedation or anaesthesia are likely to have additional needs compared with outpatients. A member of the radiology team should liaise with ward staff regarding preparation for the procedure or the requirements of the care pathway.

4.4 Day of procedure

4.4.1 When patients who are likely to receive analgesia, sedation or a general anaesthetic arrive in the radiology department they should be received into a suitable waiting area. This should be situated close to the recovery area to enable the most efficient use of nursing staff. The area should:

- be protected and quiet;
- enable identification of the patient;
- be used for countersigning the consent form;
- have staff in attendance for handover.

Compliance with the preparation checklist can be carried out and an assessment of the current status made.

4.4.2 For patients having long interventional procedures particular attention should be paid to patient comfort including the following:

- hydration—moistening the mouth with water carries little risk and increases comfort. A dehydrated patient may be at greater risk of thrombosis;
- padding for the back—many patients have osteoarthritic changes in the back and hips which can cause more discomfort than the procedure;
- support under the calves to lift heels off the table may increase comfort and reduce the need for drugs and the risk of pressure areas;
- protection of painful, ischaemic feet. It may be necessary to lift drapes off the feet or even to hang them over the edge of the table for part of a vascular procedure if ischaemic pain cannot be well-controlled;
- use of blankets to prevent hypothermia;
- if patients need to lie in oblique or prone positions extra care should be taken with comfort.

5 Consent

5.1 Local guidelines should be developed in accord with General Medical Council (GMC) policy.

5.2 In general for an elective procedure requiring sedation or anaesthesia the process of obtaining consent by providing adequate information should have been started by the requestor or in the pre-assessment phase of the patient's encounter with the radiology department. Giving information at an early stage enables the patient to think about the planned procedure and its implications. A consent form can be signed before or at the pre-assessment stage, and the radiologist can answer any further questions regarding the procedure when the patient arrives for it.

5.3 For an emergency procedure consent may have to be obtained when the patient reaches the radiology department, and this should be obtained in accordance with local protocols.

6 Monitoring

6.1 A suitably trained person must monitor patients given any analgesics, sedatives or an anaesthetic. Ideally this person will not have any other role at the time of the procedure. Although it is recognised that this is currently a difficult area for many departments, the overriding consideration must be that patient safety should not be compromised because of staffing or financial constraints.

6.2 Even if only small amounts of medication are being used, it must be remembered that idiosyncratic reactions to small doses can produce a potentially dangerous situation. Trainee radiologists, even if trained in sedation and monitoring, should not be used to monitor patients if it is to the detriment of other aspects of their radiological training.

6.3 The radiologist performing the procedure is not able to monitor the patient adequately[7] and should not be tempted to do so. It is essential that the role of the radiologist performing the procedure is separate from that of the person monitoring the level of sedation.

6.4 Valuable information can be obtained by talking with, and observation of, the patient throughout a procedure. Wincing or other evidence of pain should prompt enquiry and additional analgesia should be considered if simpler remedies are insufficient.

6.5 Whilst radiographers and healthcare assistants can give valuable help in observing patients and ensuring their comfort, they should not be expected to be responsible for the formal monitoring of the patient, unless they have been specifically trained.

6.6 In the event of an emergency rapid access to additional staff is required and the mechanism by which this is obtained should have been planned and tested.

6.7 Parameters that may be monitored are:

- oxygen saturation. The SpO_2 cannot be reliably assessed by clinical observation and all patients should have continuous pulse oximetry. The SpO_2 should be maintained at or above 95%. Routine administration of oxygen by face mask or nasal cannulae at 2–4 l/min is recommended for all patients having intravenous sedation;[9]
- heart rate;
- respiratory rate and pattern;
- blood pressure;
- level of sedation;
- discomfort—pain control, tolerance;
- perfusion—skin colour, warmth;
- hydration—infusion pumps;
- urine output (if catheterised). Consider case duration if not catheterised;
- undesirable side-effects.

6.8 An SpO_2 below 90% is dangerous and requires immediate intervention.

6.9 There should be regular assessment of blood pressure, heart rate and SpO_2. Any adverse events should be fully recorded in the patient's notes. Good documentation promotes continuity of care, improves communication among team members and provides a mechanism for audit of patient outcomes.

7 Equipment

7.1 Radiology rooms where patients are given analgesic or sedative drugs or general anaesthetics need to be adequately equipped with modern equipment for monitoring and resuscitation (see below). The equipment may be stored in an adjoining area. Limitations imposed by magnetic fields can be considerable and need to be thought through in detail (see Section 11.3—Cross-sectional imaging).

- oxygen (piped), humidifier, nitrous oxide with air (piped) for general anaesthetic. Supplemental oxygen should be used routinely in interventional procedures;[9]*
- suction (mechanical), oral suckers, catheters;*
- masks—Venti, Hudson, Laerdal, nasal cannulae;
- airways—oral, nasal, pharyngeal;
- ambu bag with mask;
- intubation instruments;
- pulse oximeter;
- anaesthetic trolley;
- blood pressure monitoring device;
- electrocardiograph;
- stethoscope;
- intravenous infusion equipment, colloidal fluids;
- analgesia/sedation, reversal, anti-convulsant, anti-emetic drugs;
- anti-anaphylaxis agents;
- defibrillator;
- tilt trolley;
- manual handling devices (e.g., patient slide);
- resuscitation trolley;*
- support for the radiographic table in the event of cardiopulmonary resuscitation being needed.

*These should be checked daily.

7.2 Patients, particularly the young and elderly, need to be kept warm and 'space blankets' and warming devices should be available.

8 Staffing

8.1 Where a radiology department is likely to need anaesthetic assistance on a regular basis, it is recommended that there is a named anaesthetist who should develop a special interest in radiological needs and be a source of expertise for their radiological and anaesthetic colleagues.

8.2 All staff need to be adequately trained and have a clear understanding of their role.

8.3 Only a minority of interventional procedures are performed outside normal departmental hours, but these patients are likely to be among the sickest patients treated. Deaths after intervention are, not surprisingly, highest in patients treated urgently or as an emergency.[7] It is essential that the daytime standards of care are not compromised for these patients. The same type and number of staff should be available for out-of-hours procedures, as adequate staffing is generally the most critical issue.[10] Each department must have a written policy for out-of-hours activity which is agreed by radiologists, radiographers, nurses, anaesthetists and the risk management team.

9 Space Requirements

9.1   Procedure rooms must be large enough to accommodate an anaesthetic machine and the personnel required in the event of a full-scale resuscitation being necessary.

9.2   All radiology departments using sedation or anaesthesia are recommended to have a recovery area within the department, staffed by radiology nurses, which can serve patients from interventional rooms, computed tomography (CT), magnetic resonance imaging (MRI) etc. The area should be quiet, warm and easily accessible to the nursing staff and close to the areas from which patients are being received. Within this area should be the same equipment as listed above for the procedure rooms.

9.3   Patients should be nursed on tipping trolleys with chairs available for the mobilisation phase of recovery if appropriate.

9.4   Rarely, patients will need to be transferred from the radiology room directly to an intensive care or high dependency bed. This possibility should be allowed for in the calculation of the requirement for these beds, especially in hospitals performing large numbers of procedures on very sick patients.

10 Patient Recovery, Transfer and Discharge

10.1 The monitoring started during the procedure should be continued through recovery until discharge criteria are met. Recovery criteria for different destinations should be developed and will include:

- intact airway, intact cough reflex;
- awake, alert and aware of surroundings;
- acceptable level of comfort;
- skin warm, dry;
- wound site dry/intact;
- haemodynamically stable compared with pre-procedure baseline blood pressure and pulse, pO_2 saturation > 95%;
- post-procedure drugs administered or prescribed;
- notes completed;
- appropriately trained escort available;
- adult supervision available for 24 h;
- handover between staff;
- outpatient appointment arranged if appropriate;
- post-procedure advice and instructions given.

10.2 The 'post-procedure' instructions should include:

- advice, both written and oral, about whom to contact if the patient feels unwell during the next 24 h. Patients should be advised against driving for 24 h;
- information on side-effects which commonly include a dry mouth, drowsiness, and an inability to perform complex tasks. Potentially dangerous occupations are best avoided for 24 h when sedative or anaesthetic drugs have been used;
- any activity which might be impaired by the residual effects of the drugs e.g., signing documents, should be avoided for 24 h.

10.3 If the patient does not meet the discharge criteria, the radiologist or anaesthetist must be notified and further instructions sought.

10.4 If the patient needs to be transferred elsewhere in the hospital while still sedated or anaesthetised they will need to be accompanied by suitable staff, and the hospital criteria for such a move should be met.

11 Subspecialty Considerations

11.1 Paediatrics

11.1.1 Definitions

The terms *analgesia* and *anaesthesia* have been defined in Section 3 and apply equally to adults and children. For children undergoing radiological examinations a deeper level of sedation is generally necessary such that the child remains asleep during the entire procedure. In these circumstances children are not expected to be able to respond to verbal stimuli.

Sedation at this level in children produces a state of depression of the nervous system such that the patient is not easily roused (by painless stimuli such as noise or movement) but which has a safety margin wide enough to render the loss of airway and breathing reflexes unlikely. No airway interventions should be required but those administering this type of sedation must be skilled in advanced paediatric airway management and life support.

11.1.2 General considerations

- Many children understand what is required of them when undergoing a radiological procedure. Anxiety and fear can be allayed by a kind and sympathetic approach from staff with paediatric expertise, thus often avoiding the need for sedation or anaesthesia.

- The environment should be suitable for children. The reassuring presence of a parent is also beneficial and should be encouraged. Newborn babies and infants under 4 months of age will tend to sleep naturally if warm and recently fed. Encouraging sleep deprivation before imaging may improve success, with or without sedation.

- For other children, however, all but the briefest radiological procedure can be frightening and distressing. Young children, in particular, find it difficult to be still even for short periods. It is inevitable that the need for general anaesthesia or sedation will be greater in children than in adults undergoing radiological examinations.

- It is strongly recommended that there is close collaboration between the radiology department and the local paediatric anaesthetic department when designing protocols for the sedation of children in radiology. The concept and practice of nurse-led sedation, whereby nurses trained in advanced paediatric life support have in essence sole responsibility for the sedation of children, is relatively new.[11] Where this model is in place, it is essential that there is close collaboration, support and regular training from the paediatric anaesthetic department.

- Any procedure that is likely to be painful or likely to induce unpleasant autonomic reflexes must be performed under general anaesthesia. Similarly, the clinical management of a child with significant pathology such as raised intracranial pressure or congenital heart disease is optimal if the airway and ventilation are controlled as part of the anaesthetic technique.

- In addition, anaesthesia is often the best choice for children who are neurologically impaired, have global developmental delay or exhibit severe disturbances of behaviour, and also where the procedure is likely to be prolonged.

- Interventional procedures in children, by their very nature, demand that analgesia be considered carefully. Sedative drugs are not analgesics and although some analgesic agents have sedative action in high doses, this comes with significant risk of unwanted respiratory and cardiovascular depression. It is inappropriate to perform anything other than the briefest interventional radiological procedure under sedation in a young child. Reduction of intussusception in small children can be performed successfully with analgesia, while sedation alone is probably best avoided.[12]

- It should be possible to regularly achieve a high successful sedation rate. Repeated failure should prompt efforts to review and improve the service. Patient variability and the need to maintain a margin of safety, however, mean that there will always be some children in whom sedation fails.

11.1.3 Parental consent

The risks and benefits of a procedure, likely outcome, and alternatives should be explained. It is important to acknowledge that sedation may fail and to explain what will happen in this event. The risks of modern anaesthesia are very low, with a risk of serious morbidity or mortality estimated at less than 1 per 250 000.[3] Information should be given about care after discharge and contact numbers provided in case of problems. It is not current practice in most UK centres to obtain written consent for the sedation of children but this may change in the future.[3]

11.1.4 Environment

The facilities for children should be safe, secure and child-friendly. Ideally, they should be separate from adult services, at least in time if not also in location. The provision of designated lists solely for children is encouraged. Careful consideration should be given to the location in which children are sedated if this is not within the radiology department: it is undesirable to transport sedated children for large distances.

11.1.5 Equipment

The facilities required for the safe administration of anaesthesia and sedation are identical. A full range of paediatric equipment is necessary.

11.1.6 Fasting guidelines

With the exception of neonates and infants under 4 months of age who may sleep naturally if recently fed, all children should be fasted before sedation or general anaesthesia. This means 6 h for solids or formula milk, 4 h for breast milk, and 2 h for clear fluids. Oral contrast for bowel opacification in CT, e.g., diluted Iohexol or Iopamidol, may be regarded as a 'clear fluid'. Prolonged starvation times should be avoided as this leads to considerable distress and adversely affects the success of sedation. It may be necessary to 'prescribe' a drink of clear fluid if there is a delay of more than 2 h.

11.1.7 Techniques

There is no ideal sedative agent in children. Some children find the disinhibition caused by sedation very distressing. This effect is largely unpredictable and is a recognised cause of 'failed sedation'. Most oral sedative drugs have relatively low potency with a slow onset and prolonged duration of action. There is always a danger that the depth of sedation will increase as absorption continues, and that the duration of sedation will significantly outlast that of the procedure. Monitoring should therefore continue until the child is ready for discharge.

Accepted criteria for discharge demand that, 2 h after sedation, the child should be easily roused, able to drink unassisted, be pain free and that the parent/carer has received relevant instructions.

The following are examples of orally administered sedative drugs that are commonly used to sedate children for radiological imaging, alternatives are available.

- *Chloral hydrate*, or its active metabolite Trichlofos, is an example of a sedative drug that has been used for many years in infants and children over 15 kg in weight or under 2 years of age. Side-effects are few when given in a single dose orally. The main disadvantage is gastric irritation, which can lead to vomiting. Dose range is 30–100 mg/kg orally with a maximum of 1 g orally. Older formularies sometimes advocate larger doses but this is not generally advisable: the duration of sedation is excessively prolonged and respiratory depression can occur.[13] Larger doses also involve giving a larger volume which increases gastric irritation.

- *Midazolam* is a more potent agent with a more rapid onset and offset of effect. The quality of anxiolysis is good although the degree of sedation is less predictable. It is bitter tasting but this can be disguised in syrup or juice, the oral dose being 0.5 mg/kg. It is suitable for children over 1 year of age undergoing brief procedures where anxiolysis or sleep is the main requirement. There is some degree of retrograde amnesia in children. Although Midazolam can also be administered intranasally (0.2 mg/kg), it stings greatly and is unpleasant.

11.1.8 General anaesthesia and intravenous sedation

These should be administered by an anaesthetist. Detailed descriptions of techniques are outside the scope of this publication. The intravenous anaesthetics Ketamine, Propofol, Thiopentone, and inhalational anaesthetic agents must not be administered by anyone other than an anaesthetist.

Fentanyl and morphine have potent respiratory depressant action, particularly in combination with other sedative agents. If, in a child, a procedure is painful enough to require these drugs, it is likely that general anaesthesia is required. Although inhalation of nitrous oxide in oxygen is safe and effective in children for brief painful procedures, it is unlikely that this will provide appropriate conditions for most radiological procedures. The advice of colleagues in the anaesthetic department should be sought if there is doubt.

Combinations of oral sedatives have had historical popularity, but it should be remembered that their perceived benefits of enhanced and greater predictability are directly attributable to additive and synergistic pharmacological effects.

11.1.9 Analgesia

Simple analgesics (non-steroidal anti-inflammatory agents or paracetamol) are very effective in children. They may be given up to 1 h before a procedure as well as afterwards. Local anaesthetic agents should be infiltrated wherever indicated.

11.2 Adult interventional radiology

11.2.1 Definition

This section covers diagnostic and interventional vascular radiology procedures and interventional non-vascular procedures. Cardiac radiology has been excluded because it has markedly different needs to non-cardiac radiology and is performed mostly by cardiologists.

11.2.2 Pre-assessment

The generic guidelines should be followed. Before an interventional procedure of the head and neck vessels, a neurological assessment is advised. These assessments should be repeated after the procedure.

11.2.3 Analgesia

Whilst some vascular procedures cause little pain, some do require sedation and analgesia. Embolization of organs and tumours may cause pain which may be severe. Patients should be warned of this and its likely duration when consent is obtained. Patient controlled analgesia may be useful for post-procedural pain. Non-vascular procedures, particularly hepatobiliary and renal intervention, tend to cause more pain than vascular intervention, and in most cases it is inappropriate to undertake them without sedation and analgesia administered by an appropriately trained heathcare professional with the appropriate level of monitoring. A planned approach with an anaesthetist, perhaps considering regional anaesthesia, may be required. Identified anaesthetist time or defined sessions should be available if required.

11.2.4 General anaesthesia

General anaesthesia is infrequently required for adult vascular diagnostic and interventional procedures. Indications for general anaesthesia include:

- patients with uncontrollable pain or severe systemic disease who will not be able to stay still;
- patients with impaired understanding of the procedure or those who cannot cooperate;
- the need for very long procedures;
- very painful procedures.

Regional, spinal or epidural anaesthesia may be used for some interventional procedures.

In neuroradiology many patients require general anaesthesia for arterial and venous diagnostic and therapeutic procedures. Identified anaesthetists and anaesthetic time is necessary in this subspecialty.

11.3 Cross-sectional imaging

11.3.1 Cross-sectional imaging techniques are relatively pain free and the need to use sedation for adult patients is infrequent. With the introduction of high speed multi-slice CT, this need should be further reduced. There are, however, a group of patients who find the narrow bore of the magnet in MRI a claustrophobic environment and require sedation to tolerate the procedure.

11.3.2 Patients with certain neurological disorders have involuntary movements which may need to be suppressed so that a scan can be obtained. Adult patients who are unable to co-operate with the procedure due to confusion complicating an acute illness or secondary to long-term mental disability present a further problem. If they require sedation, appropriate consent needs to be obtained according to the hospital guidelines. In this situation the level of sedation may be such that it is advisable that an anaesthetist is present to administer the appropriate agent and supervise during the procedure.

11.3.3 Other patients, such as those with rheumatoid arthritis, may be unable to lie flat or still for the length of time the examination takes. The need for sedation and anaesthesia must be considered when an MRI unit is being planned because of the constraints imposed by the magnetic field.

11.3.4 To reduce the need for sedation in patients suffering from claustrophobia or anxiety, prone positioning can be helpful.

11.3.5 Some patients are able to tolerate the procedure following an oral sedative and should be encouraged to do so. Those choosing oral sedation should arrive 1.5 h before the procedure and be fasting.

11.4 Patient safety during procedure

11.4.1 In the case of magnetic resonance (MR) there should be a recognised protocol for removing the patient from the magnet and summoning the emergency resuscitation team.

11.4.2 The hospital resuscitation team needs to know where the MR unit is located.

11.4.3 The MR examination room should be designed so that the patient table can be rapidly removed from the magnetic environment and the patient transferred to an appropriately designated resuscitation area in close proximity to the MR examination room.

11.5 Equipment for MRI[14]

11.5.1 Anaesthetic equipment that is used in the scanning room must be MRI compatible i.e., presenting no hazard to patients or personnel when it is taken into the MR scanning room. MR compatible equipment is magnetic resonance safe, functions normally in the MR environment, and does not interfere with the correct operation of the MRI equipment providing instructions regarding its proper use are followed.

11.5.2 MR compatible equipment must be easily distinguishable from standard equipment. The hazards associated with using the wrong equipment include the projectile effect, burns and malfunction, e.g., non-MR compatible syringe drivers may deliver drugs incorrectly.

11.5.3 Monitoring of patients during anaesthesia and sedation in the magnet bore requires MR compatible monitoring equipment and must comply with minimum monitoring standards. A remote monitoring facility should be available to allow the sedationist/anaesthetic team to remain outside the scanning room once the patient is settled. This also enables the staff to be away from the noise of the MRI machine and repeated exposure to the strong magnetic field.

11.5.4 MR compatible pulse oximeters must use fibre-optic cabling to avoid burns and special electrocardiograph electrodes are needed. Padding should be placed between cables and the patient's skin and cables should not be allowed to form loops within the scanner (loops can induce current and hence burn the patient). The responsibility for the safe placement of MR monitoring equipment should be allocated to a small number of personnel who understand the problems and risks.

11.6 CT and MRI with the severely ill patient

Patients transferred from the emergency room or intensive care unit to radiology require full monitoring by an anaesthetist during transfer as well as during the imaging investigation. The radiology department is a potentially dangerous place for the emergency patient. Patients for these procedures should not be moved to radiology until they are stable unless the cause of that instability requires immediate diagnosis to enable treatment to be undertaken. Examples of the latter might include the requirement for control of blood loss, or the dispersal and lysis of a massive pulmonary embolus. Movement around the hospital of recently admitted trauma, or seriously ill patients for investigation should be as rigorously planned as inter-hospital transfer. The UK Intensive Care Society guidelines for transport of the critically ill adult, can be applied equally to the intra-hospital transfer of patients from the emergency room or ICU, to the department of radiology.[15]

11.6.1 Intensive care patients and MRI

It is possible to examine intensive care unit patients with MRI, but it needs planning and plenty of time. The main problems are caused by the number of lines and infusion pumps attached to the patient. These should be disconnected unless absolutely essential. Those infusions that must be continued need extensions of adequate length to keep the pumps outside the 30 gauss line as pumps will malfunction above this field strength.

All patients referred for MR procedures with cardiovascular catheters and accessories that have internally or externally positioned conductive wires or similar components should not undergo MRI, unless the catheter is removed, because of the risk of excessive heating in the wires.

The management of anaesthesia, and intensive care patients in MRI is a skilled and specialist area. It should not be undertaken by an anaesthestist or intensivist who has not received appropriate training, and who has not had experience of working in this environment.

12 Training and Continuing Professional Development

12.1 Training

12.1.1 Training in safe analgesia and sedation practice has not featured formally in the training of most radiologists to date and should now be included in the specialist registrar training curricula. Trainees should have teaching about sedation and analgesia when they are introduced to vascular, interventional and cross-sectional radiology. Specialist registrar training should include resuscitation. Knowledge of the essential elements of safe practice should include:

- understanding relevant applied pharmacology and physiology;
- monitoring parameters and equipment;
- 'reversal' drugs;
- basic life support measures.

Consideration should be given to testing these during the FRCR examination

12.1.2 Between them, the radiology team needs to be able to recognise common arrythmias and know how to treat them if required.

12.1.3 Appropriate life support training is mandatory for all staff working with sedated or anaesthetised patients. Staff should be familiar with the location of call buttons in all rooms where such patients are treated and know where resuscitation equipment is kept.

12.1.4 For satisfactory continued professional development, refresher lectures on sedation and analgesia should be included in postgraduate courses, especially for interventional radiologists, but also for paediatric and cross-sectional radiologists. Computer-based learning packages can be an effective way for wide dissemination of such instruction.[16]

12.1.5 Continuing medical education points could be awarded for visiting colleagues to learn new techniques or update their knowledge on existing practices. Where 'hub and spoke' relationships exist between large and smaller departments, there should be educational interchange between them to encourage uniform good practice.

12.2 Nursing staff skills

Radiology department nurses looking after patients having analgesia, sedation or general anaesthetics need to be trained and competent in:

- administration of analgesia/sedation/reversal agents;
- pharmacology of medications/reactions;
- airway management, advanced life support training;
- respiratory functions (oxygen delivery, transport, uptake);
- function of oxygen, monitoring equipment, Entonox (if used);
- data interpretation, cardiac arrhythmias;
- relevant anatomy and physiology;
- function of infusion devices and knowledge of infusion fluids;
- cannulation skills;
- haemostasis.

13 Audit

13.1 As part of good clinical governance, radiology departments should liase with their anaesthetic colleagues to perform periodic audits of the effectiveness of their arrangements for all aspects of analgesia, sedation and anaesthesia. Subjects to study include:[17]

- what patients think of the information they were given;
- the frequency and outcome of complications/unplanned events/critical incidents;
- the frequency of unplanned admission to a ward or intensive care;
- the adequacy of analgesia and sedation;
- abandoned procedures;
- calls for anaesthetic help—urgent or emergency;
- resuscitation competence of key staff;
- presence of local protocols and guidelines;
- morbidity and mortality.

13.2 It is to be hoped that improved practice has developed in UK radiology departments since a report in 1993 showed *inter alia* limited use of monitoring and infrequent use of additional oxygen.[18]

13.3 The outcomes of audit may provide justification for changes in practice or further resources.

14 Revalidation

14.1   Revalidation of doctors will be based on the results of annual appraisals so radiologists need to collect audit results and other data which will contribute to satisfactory appraisals. It will be important for radiologists to be able to show competence and adequate performance in the practice of sedation and analgesia, if it is relevant to their practice, as part of revalidation.

Approved by the Board of the Faculty of Clinical Radiology: 4 July 2003
Approved by Council 25 July 2003
BFCR(03)4

References

1   Joint Publication The Royal College of Radiologists/The Royal College of Anaesthetists (1992) *Sedation and Anaesthesia in Radiology*. London: The Royal College of Radiologists

2   Intercollegiate Working Party chaired by the Royal College of Anaesthetists (2001) *Implementing and Ensuring Safe Sedation Practice for Healthcare Procedures in Adults*. Report available from the Royal College of Anaesthetists

3   Scottish Intercollegiate Guidelines Network (2002) *Safe Sedation of Children Undergoing Diagnostic and Therapeutic Procedures*. (www.sign.ac.uk)

4   Association of Anaesthetists of Great Britain and Ireland (2002) *Provision of Anaesthetic Services in Magnetic Resonance Units*. London: Association of Great Britain and Ireland (www.aagbi.org)

5   Watkinson AF, Francis IS, Torrie P, Platts AD (2002) The role of anaesthesia in interventional radiology *Br J Radiol* **75**:105–106

6   Mueller PR, Biswal S, Halpern EF, Kaufman JA, Lee MJ (2000) Interventional radiologic procedures: patient anxiety, perception of pain, understanding of procedure, and satisfaction with medication – a prospective study. *Radiology* **215**(3):684–688

7   National Confidential Enquiry into Perioperative Deaths (2000) *Interventional Vascular Radiology and Interventional Neurovascular Radiology*. London: NCEPOD

8   The Wylie Report: Report of the Working Party on Training in Dental Anaesthesia (1981) *Br Dental J* **151**:385–388

9   Rigg J, Watt T, Tweedle DEF, Martin DF (1991) Abolition of hypoxia during ERCP with pre-oxygenation. *Gut* **32**:A567

10 The Royal College of Radiologists (2001) *Guidelines for Nursing Care in Interventional Radiology* BFCR(01)3. London: The Royal College of Radiologists

11 Sury MRJ, Hatch DJ, Deeley T, Dicks-Mireaux C, Chong WK (1999) Development of a nurse-led sedation service for paediatric magnetic resonance imaging. *Lancet* **353**:1667–1671

12 Rosenfeld K, McHugh K (1999) Survey of intussusception reduction in England, Scotland and Wales – how and why we could do better. *Clin Radiol* **54**(7):452–458

13 Keengwe IN, Hegde S, Dearlove O, Wilson B, Yates, RW, Sharples A (1999) Structured sedation programme for magnetic resonance imaging examination in children. *Anaesthesia* **54**: 1069–1072

14 The Royal College of Anaesthetists (1999) *Guidelines for the Provision of Anaesthetic Services*. London: Royal College of Anaesthetists

15 Intensive Care Society (2002) *Guidelines for the Transport of the Critically Ill Adult*. London: Intensive Care Society

16 Medina LS, Racadio JM, Schwid HA (2000) Computers in Radiology. The sedation, analgesia, and contrast media computerized simulator: a new approach to train and evaluate radiologists' responses to critical incidents. *Paediatr Radiol* **30**(5):299–305

17 Godwin R, de Lacey G, Manhire A (1996) *Clinical Audit in Radiology: 100+ Recipes*. London: The Royal College of Radiologists. ISBN 1 872599 19 2

18 McDermott VGM, Chapman ME, Gillespie I (1993) Sedation and monitoring in vascular and interventional radiology. *Br J Radiol* **66**: 667–671